A truly classic Treatise & Step-by-Step Guide to OVERCOMING Ill-Health by opening up our Heart & Mind, as well as our Spirit & Soul to Healing Ourselves thru & thru . . . . on ALL Levels . . . . Charise shows us that the "Classroom" of a Life-Threatening Illness can be the Greatest Gift we can receive in teaching us to ultimately have "the most" Happy & Successful Lives possible!!!!

William E Richardson, MD

Lee   Continue to grow and strive with Sacred Tai Chi!

   Love
    Chi

HEALING GIFTS FROM OUR PLANET

A Woman's Journey to Vibrant Health
"Inside Every Seed Is A Whole Tree"

CHARISE

Copyright © 2012 by CHARISE.

ISBN:	Softcover	978-1-4691-9187-4
	Ebook	978-1-4691-9188-1

All rights reserved. No part of this book may be reproduced or transmitted in any form or by any means, electronic or mechanical, including photocopying, recording, or by any information storage and retrieval system, without permission in writing from the copyright owner.

The information presented in this book is for educational purposes only. This information is not intended to diagnose, mitigate, cure or prevent any disease, medical, or psychological condition or replace the advice of a qualified health care professional. The author, physicians, practitioners, characters, and publisher of this book and their agents assume no responsibility/liability for the misuse of the content within this text. How you the reader, use this information is solely your responsibility.

This book was printed in the United States of America.

Editor: Lynn Stratton
Glossary Tenanche Rosegolden

To order additional copies of this book, contact:
Xlibris Corporation
1-888-795-4274
www.Xlibris.com
Orders@Xlibris.com

CONTENTS

Foreword 9
Introduction   Building a Bridge from Sickness to Health 11

Chapter 1:   Crossing The Bridge 13
Chapter 2:   The Power of Awareness 15
Chapter 3:   Compromising Wealth For Health 19
Chapter 4:   The I.V. Experience: An Uphill Battle 21
Chapter 5:   Returning To Atlanta 24
Chapter 6:   What Can I Eat, and Is it Going To Taste Good? 28
Chapter 7:   Changing Your Environment: Making Your Space
             a Healing Place Conducive to Wellness 30
Chapter 8:   Food Is Everything You Think:
             Change Your Thinking and Change Your World 32
Chapter 9:   Excuses, Attachments, and Cheeta Willies:
             Organic Foods Cost Too Much 34
Chapter 10: Ahimki Blessing: Vibrations of Wellness 36
Chapter 11: Pushing Through The Pain:
             My Departure from Work and a Higher Calling 39
Chapter 12: Receiving the Dao, and Finally Seeing "The Way" 41
Chapter 13: The Accident: Using My Gifts 44
Chapter 14: Returning to Tai Chi 46
Chapter 15: Tai Chi For Real: Getting My Mojo Back 48
Chapter 16: The Sun (Ra): Standing and Sitting in the Light 50
Chapter 17: Good Night: Catching some *Zzzzzzzz's*. 52
Chapter 18: Tweaking The Program 54
Chapter 19: Forgiving Everyone Means Forgiving Yourself 57
Chapter 20: Pulling It All Together 59
Chapter 21: Crossing The Finish Line: Your Investment in Yourself 61

Summing it Up 63
Tai Chi/Qi Gong Update 65
Glossary 67

Acknowledgements

This book is dedicated to my mother, Dr. Rachel Poole, Ph.D. Nurse, and my father, Dr. Marion L. Poole, ED.D, who came together and gifted me physical life. They both were both healer and teacher to me. Thanks, Mom and Dad, for gifting me your DNA.

I also dedicate this book to my two children Aisha and EJ, through whom I now not understand but innerstand what true unconditional love is and who made me stretch my limits multidimensionally since the day they were each conceived. You have brought profound joy into my life that I would have never known or even imagined. Thank you.

To my two sisters, M L Poole and Tenanche Rose Golden: Understanding and wisdom always departed from your lips, even when I didn't want it to. I love you both.

To my favorite Aunt Bernice: You always believed in me no matter what, and you always told it like it TIS.

To my very best friend, Darryl Spencer, who always stood beside me and guided me through many loving and painful years. You've always imparted love, compassion, and spiritual wisdom. Thank you for always helping to pick me up when I fell.

Divine Spirit and Light, I am, now and forevermore, eternally grateful.

To Richard Oshetoye, who helped me to get organized: You pushed me to finish this book to get it in the hands of so many hue-mans. You said, "Get it done! A lot of people are in need of this information that only you can give." Thank you, my best friend as well.

To all of the unnamed relatives, friends and divine souls of light who have impacted my life. You know who you are. I thank you.

My special thanks goes out to the ancestors, archangels and spirit guides without whom none of this would have been possible: Standing and walking with me always and helping to awaken the Spirit in me.

Most profound thanks to God/Goddess, The Most High and Ultimate One, who granted me Grace and not only a first, but a second chance at life in this lifetime to even become immortal, which I now choose to be.

With Much Humility and Gratitude,

Hotep

Foreword

By William E Richardson, MD . . . Medical Director of
The American Clinics for Preventive Medicine, Inc.
www.acpm.net

In over 35 Years of Education, Training & extensive Experience in Medicine and the Healing Arts, I have seen a Multitude of my Patients overcome almost every Illness, Disease & Condi-tion known to Mankind!!!! Also, I have unfortunately seen patients Defeated by "these same"
Health Challenges. Often, I have pondered & wondered . . . . What is "the Difference" between
One who Overcomes Illness and One who does NOT????
Is "the Difference":

- Lack, Limitation & Poverty
- Difficult Circumstances
- "Severity" of their Condition
- Lack of Support
- Lack of Knowledge

While "these Factors" certainly do have an impact on how we need to Proceed in our Healing Quest; we must also Remember & Utilize the Divine UNIVERSAL Laws that give us the Knowledge, Motivation, Inspiration & unlimited Resources that can Completely Empower Us to OVERCOME Anything!!!!

★

    I Applaud Charise as she shares her Tremendous Healing Journey that called on her to Learn, Apply & Master the Universal Laws, Tools & Energies that are available to Us all.

    Finally, while Charise encourages us to seek all kinds of Healing Techniques possible, she also makes it very clear that there is no Doctor, Bottle of Pills, Priest, Preacher, Guru or anything else that can give you Complete Healing except the GOD within You!!!!

    I found her Book "Healing GIFTS from our Planet" to be an Outstanding Healing Guide that is Well-Written, Stimulating & Engaging. I Trust & Pray that we all embrace & utilize the "Gifts" we have all been given in this Wonderful Work.

Introduction

Building a Bridge from Sickness to Health

So you wake up one day and realize you don't feel well, haven't felt well in ages.

You start looking for answers with little success. You go from doctor to doctor only for them to tell you (after a series of tests) that they can't find anything wrong with you. Perhaps they even say it's all in your head.

Then you start looking up your symptoms online. You search and search, only to find myriad diseases and illnesses that *could* be your problem. And you realize that part of you wants to find an illness, but another part of you doesn't.

But you may feel you have little choice in the matter because you just aren't feeling well—but that is just plain unacceptable. So you hope and pray in your conscious and unconscious mind that you find something that is not really serious.

Your time is limited, of course, because you have to go to work in the morning, which you dread because you know you'll probably wake up tired. And if you're not tired, then maybe you're nauseated, or shaky, or you're constipated or have diarrhea.

Waking up and just feeling tired, well, that seems like a good day in comparison. And you think, Good day? Since when is *that* normal?

This is how I lived, or at least existed, for almost two years. Now, I don't know about you, but I want to feel *alive*. I want to feel healthy and vibrant. I don't want mediocre days, I want great days, everyday.

Feeling fatigued, day in and day out, should not be the only option.

⭐

    This is how I felt during those two years, and this book is about what I did about it.

    Chinese medicine tells us, "There is no such thing as an incurable disease," and through my journey, I have found that it is true.

Chapter 1

Crossing The Bridge

When I first became ill, I felt weak, tired, and nauseated. I wasn't able to keep a lot of foods down. Sometimes I'd even get an unexplained rash. In fact, my body was so full of surprises that I had no idea which particular ailment it was going to manifest on any day.

So I went from doctor to doctor: primary care physician, neurologist, dermatologist, ophthalmologist, gynecologist, eye and ear doctors . . . so many I can't even remember them all or the number of visits I'd had with each one.

And each one would ask me what the others had said, and then they always came up with the same conclusion: that everything was normal. My cholesterol was a little high, but other than that, I was normal.

I was glad to know that, but what could it be that was depleting my strength and vitality and making me nauseated? I was also slipping in mental sharpness, which was very unusual for me because my memory had always been nearly perfect. Thank goodness it never affected my ability to perform at work, but everything I did took more effort to complete.

After spiraling downhill for about two years and feeling like a hamster on an ever-turning wheel, I decided to travel back to my hometown several states away to revisit a naturopath, I had seen many years ago. I'll just call him Dr T. I hadn't seen him in about five years, having been so involved in my career in Georgia. But Dr. T always had the answers I needed, and I knew that if he didn't know what was going on, probably nobody did.

I knew I had to see him. But when I called to make my appointment, the nurse said he would not be available for about four more months.

★

I thought, Since when does my doctor become unavailable to me? So I proceeded to explain my urgency to the nurse.

And the nurse explained to me that Dr. T, had decided after about thirty years to also become an M.D. and was about two months into his six-month residency at a local hospital.

Compassionately, the nurse said she would schedule an appointment for me four months out so that I would be one of his first patients when he returned to his practice. Well, I was glad to get the appointment, of course, but I was disappointed, to say the least.

My health was steadily going downhill, and I didn't know why. I didn't even know if I would survive long enough to see him.

So the next several months felt like a century. I decided to continue doctor-hunting and muddled through physician after physician, even revisiting some of the ones I had seen before. One of them thought I was making things up, and I wished I were. I would go home at night from work and have tremors, along with the nausea, diarrhea and headaches. I could hardly focus on anything except the illness in my body. Even my brain hurt.

And so my quest continued.

Chapter 2

The Power of Awareness

During this time, I felt very confused. I was still working 10- to12-hour days, six to seven days a week, and going home exhausted every night. But I still searched online, reading about symptoms and trying to come up with some sort of diagnosis on my own.

But as puzzling as it was to me, it was even more puzzling to the doctors, every one that I visited. I went to my PCP again, revisited my gynecologist, my ENT physicians, dermatologist and ophthalmologist, because now even my skin and my left eye hurt.

Although no one at work knew I was ill, I finally decided to ask my friend and co-worker, Michael, if he knew of a local naturopath here in Georgia. He said yes, Dr. Richardson. Well, I thought, here is a little ray of sunshine, a little ray of hope to find some answers.

I couldn't wait to see him, so I scheduled my appointment, once again looking for answers and, I hoped, a cure.

My appointment with Dr. Richardson was the following week. When I arrived at his office I was greeted by John Richardson, who is the office manager and also the Doctors brother. "Welcome, what brings you in today," he said warmly. I reluctantly began explaining my symptoms as I had done with many doctors before. He listened intensely in acknowledgement to what I was saying. Then he responded, "Well, Dr. Richardson has assisted in healing others with far worse symptoms than the ones you have. John Richardson began to give me several examples and testimonials of others who have been helped. I sat in amazement as I listened. Hope began to rise within me. Finally someone understands, I have arrived at the right place. Although I was still nervous about moving forward because this was

⭐

all still very new to me, I expressed that to him. John Richardson assured me that it was completely normal to be nervous but assured me that they could help.

Feeling a little more at ease after our conversation, I entered Dr Richardson's exam room. He greeted me warmly as well. He read over the notes that John had written and shook his head in assurance as if he had seen this kind of thing before. I found him to be very knowledgeable and personable. He explained that diet plays a key role in illness. I was relatively clueless at that time, but I didn't think I ate that badly. He was a huge light among the darkness!

He also suggested that I do a vitamin C infusion, which is vitamin C administered intravenously, to build myself up. At that point, I was willing to try just about anything, and during my consultation with him I explained as best I could some recent history. I told him I had most recently had two amalgam fillings removed and replaced with composites because of everything I'd been reading about the dangers of amalgam, or mercury, fillings.

"Ahh," he said. "You probably need to chelate." I asked him what that was, and how much it would cost.

He told me another IV in my arm would pull out the mercury and other heavy metals in my body that might be harming me, and how much it would cost. He also said most people need between eight and thirty visits for the treatment to be effective.

Well, I wasn't trying to spend that much time or money. Just fix this and I'll be on my way, I thought. Besides, I wasn't feeling entirely comfortable with that idea. The vitamin C, maybe. I told him, let's try that one first.

So, I began his protocol of Vitamin C intravenously. I showed up every week for the next two months. The treatments would have to be paid out of pocket because, as Dr Richardson explained to me, naturopaths generally don't accept insurance. However, it was still a small price to pay to get my health back.

The vitamin C infusions were extremely helpful, but I was looking for what I considered a cure. Dr. Richardson explained to me that healing takes place over time. He scheduled three one on one workshop sessions with me. In these sessions he explained to me about the body, the healing process, food consumption and nutrition and many other things. I had an opportunity to ask as many questions that I wanted. He also, gave me a twelve page diagnosis of my entire situation. I am so grateful and thanked Dr. Richardson for his insight which actually started me on my healing journey. Dr. Richardson had many of the answers I was searching for. Some which I was not yet ready to hear, like giving up chicken however, with his protocol of diet change alone, my body began to heal. I also began to feel supported going to him and The Atlanta Clinic For Preventative Medicine. Not only did I feel supported, I was armed with valuable information by way of DVD's and CD's packed with powerful healing information. For example, vegetarianism, solving digestive problems, juicing and live raw food diet, and stress management just to name a few. The education alone was in itself healing.

In the meantime, I was still searching for the answers online, and praying, I still needed more. I knew that if I was going to come out of this, it was going to have to happen soon—very soon.

During my next visit to Dr. Richardson, although supported, I explained to him how alone I felt with this illness. He called it "situational depression." As I was on my way out, his nurse, Mia, asked me if everything was all right. I told her how alone I felt in my situation and asked, "Isn't there someone else who might be going through this as well? It's hard to believe I'm the only one."

Mia said, "I know someone else with a similar condition. She lives in Atlanta, and she has similar symptoms."

I was suddenly excited. I asked who it was.

"I can't give you her name because of patient confidentiality," Mia told me. "But I will tell her you'd like to talk to her, and see what she says"

I told Mia that would be wonderful, and yes, I would like that very much.

But a week went by and I did not hear anything from Mia. Knowing about the mystery woman who lived in Atlanta with a similar illness really had me paying attention every time my phone rang—but each time, it wasn't Mia.

When I returned to Dr. Richardson's office for my next visit, Mia said, "Hey, how are you?" She told me she'd spoken with the other patient, Kelly, and that she had said it was okay to give me her contact information.

I thought, this sounds like another big break. I had a lot of questions for Kelly, and I hoped she had some answers for me.

Mia told me that Kelly was an attorney, so I tried to decide when the best time to call her would be. I wanted everything to be right when I connected with her, and, being in the travel business myself, I knew that timing was everything.

⭐

I decided to wait until the weekend. When I called Kelly that Saturday, she was so very warm and friendly. Our exchange was informative, but light.

When I asked her how she could be so calm about the illness we seemed to share, why she wasn't obsessed about it, as I was, she explained that she attended a POA workshop.

I asked her what that was. "Power of Awareness," she said. "And it was the one thing that turned everything around."

I asked her where I could find one, and how much it cost—and when she told me, I said, "Oh, I can't afford that!" I explained to her how much I was already paying Dr. Richardson, and that it was on top of the original consultation fee.

Kelly asked me how much I could afford, and suggested an amount. I hesitated, then said, "Well, it would be a stretch, but . . ."

Kelly said, "I will foot the rest for you because I know it will help you. Just promise me that after it is all over, you will help someone else. In other words, pay it forward."

"That's a promise," I told her.

Attending that workshop for three days was the experience of a lifetime for me.

There were about twenty of us. We laughed and cried together. I felt as if I were in a cocoon of time and space, with like-minded people, and all of us sharing and believing that we could think differently about our situations.

I became aware for the first time in my life that it is the things we tell ourselves, in our own minds, that create everything in our lives. We all were able to diminish a lot of our pain during those three days, and I sincerely appreciated my facilitator, Liana, who was absolutely fabulous.

But most of all, I thanked my new friend, Kelly, who had made it possible for me to be part of it.

Chapter 3

Compromising Wealth For Health

When my appointment finally came with Dr. T, I could hardly wait to see him. Although Dr. Richardson was handling things quite nicely, I still wanted to keep my appointment with Dr T.

I was experiencing new and distressing symptoms, like numbness in my arms and legs and feet. My eyes had also become progressively more sensitive to light. I was more tired than ever, and now my hair was thinning.

I was hoping Dr. T had some answers for me.

After I signed in, the receptionist took me back to the examining room.

The nurse came in first to do the initial intake, which lasted about thirty minutes, and then she left.

Not long afterward, Dr. T entered the exam room. "Hi," he said. "Where have you been?"

I laughed. "Me? Where have *you* been? I've been trying to get to you in like forever—and you decide to become an M.D. after all these years and disappear on me when I come down with something that no one can figure out."

He sat down in the examining room chair while I sat on the table, as if we were going to have a little fireside chat. Then, looking at me over his wire-rimmed glasses, he began to ask me a series of questions.

Dr. T listened although I had the feeling that he already knew what I was dealing with, but that he had to be sure. When I was done, he explained how sugar, in its many different forms, could be causing many of my symptoms. He also said that heavy metals in the body are an additional culprit. The protocol, he said, is to eliminate sugar from my diet, to build up my immune system, and to chelate the heavy metals out. There was my confirmation. Same protocol as Dr. Richardson. I now would have to make some decisions about what to do and, more importantly, how to manage it.

Dr. T recommended a high-protein, low-carbohydrate diet. "Absolutely no sugar," he said. "None."

I asked him why I couldn't eat carbohydrates. "Carbs turn into sugar in the body," he said.

"You mean no more potatoes?" I said, thinking out loud.

"Nope," he said.

Well, I said, "Okay, I'll do it!" I decided right then and there that I was willing to do whatever it took to get well. I was sick and tired, beyond sick and tired, of being sick.

Dr. T also recommended vitamin C infusion and chelation treatments and said that most people have candida problems and heavy metal toxicity. "This is why I also recommend the chelation treatments to pull out the heavy metals," he said. "We can test you for those too, if you want."

I told him I'd been tested recently for heavy metals about a month before, but that I had not gotten my results back yet.

"You also need to be on a regimen of vitamins to build yourself up in between your IV treatments," he went on to say.

I thought, Wow, how much is all this going to cost me? And how long will it last? I asked him.

"It's going to be awhile," he said. "But remember, it took you a while to get sick, so it's going to take you some time to get well."

"Anything," I said. I was willing to do almost anything legally and morally possible to keep the ball from rolling farther downhill and picking up speed. It sounded like an expensive endeavor, but I knew that I had to now trade my wealth for my health.

Chapter 4

The I.V. Experience: An Uphill Battle

When we were done going over my diagnosis, suggestions and recommendations, Dr. T. hugged me and sent me to the IV room for my first treatment.

In the treatment room, Joan, the head nurse, welcomed me. "Do you want your vitamin C drip first, to build you up before we take you down with the chelation?"

I had no idea what that meant, but I told her it sounded like a good idea. She said okay and proceeded to place the intravenous line into my arm. I wasn't sure what to expect, but I knew it had to be better than what I was currently experiencing.

I was dying, I knew that. I was suffering a slow, critical deterioration in my health. So, bring on the IVs, I thought.

I sat there for about two and a half hours that first session. I felt a little dizzy, but the nurses said that was normal.

When I left the office, I got into my car and drove to my mother's home, where I was staying, about an hour away. But about thirty minutes into my drive, I felt as if my equilibrium was slightly off. About two hours after my arrival at her home, I began to have terrible tremors, nausea, and vomiting, and then I was shocked to realize a urinary tract infection had also settled in. My body was in some sort of distress that I had not known before. I thought I was supposed to feel better, not worse.

I didn't realize it then, but know now, that I was experiencing my first die-off symptoms from the yeast in my body being killed, and my body's reaction as the heavy metals were being excreted from my body.

★

In a panic, I called Dr. T's emergency number and, with heart palpitations and tears in my eyes, I left a message. Within ten minutes, he called me back. He explained to me (again, as he had done in his office) what was happening, and told me what supplements to take.

But I didn't have any. At the end of my treatment earlier that day, I had not purchased the supplements that would sustain me in between visits. I'd planned on getting them the following day, since I had three appointments scheduled three days in a row.

Dr. T comforted me by explaining what was taking place, assuring me that I would get through this episode and saying he would see me again tomorrow.

I immediately lay down and tried to sleep it off, hoping I would survive to see him again the next day.

The next morning, I was weak and still nauseated, but I didn't feel nearly as bad as I did the night before. So, I got myself up like a woman on a mission, got into my rental car and drove back to his office for my appointment.

When he saw me, he said, "Well, how are you doing today?"

"Better than last night," I said.

"Yeah, that chelation can do that to you, and, as you heal, you may experience that kind of stuff from time to time."

I said, "Well, I'll do whatever it takes."

He smiled at me. "And one more thing, that diet of high protein and low carbs is going to make you lose a lot of weight."

"What?"

"Yep" he said. "But I wouldn't worry about that. You'll be providing your body all the nutrients that it needs, especially with the leafy greens and the vitamins you'll be taking."

I didn't want to lose any weight. I was happy with my current weight, about 135 pounds, and in proportion to my height of about 5 feet 6.

Dr. T. saw the look on my face. "Well, the alternative—" he started to say, but I stopped him.

"Okay, I'll do it. And is there anything else I should know that you haven't told me?"

He looked up from writing on my chart with a slight smile and said, "No, I'll see you again tomorrow, go on over to Chelation."

As I found myself heading back to the room that had made me violently ill the previous day, I felt like I was going back into a dungeon. Yesterday's visit there had made me so ill, I wanted to jump out of my skin or, at the least, run out of there and never come back.

But where was I to go? I'd only be running away from myself. Dr. T had always helped me heal in the past. So, knowing it was the right thing to do, I entered the room marked *Chelation Therapy*.

The nurses, as usual, were all pleasant, kind, and professional, which made the experience much more palatable. I figured that if I was going to expire, I'd rather go this way, instead of flying back to Atlanta without much family and feeling alone.

I also felt like I was in a boat without a paddle. At least here in my hometown, I was among loved ones who cared about me, and with my doctor, whom I trusted. Besides, he and Dr Richardson were the only one who had answers, and I had a lot of questions. I had to accept that, right then, my questions could not all be answered. I was just getting used to the fact that I was sick, really sick, that I had to get stuck with another IV and hope that it did not make me as ill as it had the day before.

I sat in the comfortable lounge chair in the chelation room watching the nurses buzz by and observed the other patients being treated. At least I now felt like my little boat had a paddle, even though I was paddling upstream.

I'm not going to lie, I was beyond scared; in fact, I was terrified. But I allowed the IV solution to enter my arm. It was not quite as bad the second time, and when it was over, I got up, made sure I had all the necessary supplements this time, paid my bill, and walked out again. And I prayed that it would be easier this time.

Chapter 5

Returning To Atlanta

After the third day of treatment at Dr. T's, I returned to Atlanta and my job.

I didn't feel a whole lot different, but I did feel a little more balanced, although only slightly. But one important change that made me feel better was the fact that at least now I knew what I was dealing with.

As I mentioned earlier, about a year before I became so ill, I'd had some dental work done. I've always had pretty decent teeth, but there was an amalgam filling that I'd had removed because I'd heard that it was unhealthy to have that stuff in your mouth. And besides, the white composites look better. (Okay, I was a little vain, I admit.)

Well, that vanity cost me. Amalgam fillings are made up of deadly mercury—you know, the same stuff they put into thermometers. I believe that the mercury had leaked into my body, and that had been confirmed by the heavy metal test that Dr. Richardson had done.

Ugh, I thought. No wonder I was sick!

I began feverishly to research all of this stuff on my own, trying to find out how to proceed from there. I stayed up late and spent every free moment when I wasn't working looking for more information on my condition.

Both Dr's had advised me to eat high protein and low carbohydrates. Okay, back to basics, I thought. Learn all the foods that are carbs and which ones are proteins. Well, I found out soon enough that this information was critical for me, because most of the foods I had been eating were carbs.

Immediately, I made the switch, only to find out that the decision was easy, but implementing it was not—at least, not at first. It took me several months to really get it right. I had to really learn how to read food labels.

(By the way, most of the food I eat now doesn't come with labels, because I buy mostly fresh, organic vegetables, minimal fresh organic fruit, some fresh wild-caught fish—no bottom feeders—and organic eggs.)

Also, for breakfast every morning for the next two and a half years, I ate raw eggs. Okay, it's not as gross as it sounds. I'd make a raw egg smoothie in the morning (you'll find the recipe at the end of this chapter). I discovered that an organic, cage-free, hormone-free, antibiotic-free egg is an almost-perfect food. I also discovered that our bodies are designed to run on fat, the good kind, like organic cold-pressed coconut oil or olive oil, or real organic butter, unsalted. (You'll find a list of some harmful fats at the end of this chapter.)

I also found out that the body needs approximately seventy-two minerals everyday, which we can get mostly from sea salt. Moreover, the human body is approximately 75-80% water, so guess what it needs the most—water! Good clean water, especially in the morning, upon rising, to break our fast from the night's rest.

I discovered so many things. But my journey to wellness was only just beginning. I promised God, The Creator and Ultimate One, that I would share as I went along, if It would allow and grant me grace to live and heal.

Information To Help Awaken Your Body's Magnificent Healing Power

This list is not all-inclusive; the manual will contain a more in-depth list of foods and how I used them. Also, unless otherwise noted, all items recommended are organic, unrefined, and cold-pressed. My motto? When in doubt, do without!

The Good Fats

Coconut oil*
Olive oil
Fish oil (Omega 3)
Palm oil
Cod liver oil
Flax oil
Seed and nut oils
Some animal fat, used sparingly
Organic, unsalted butter in small amounts

The Bad Fats

All hydrogenated oils
Soy, corn and safflower oils
Cottonseed oil
Canola oil
Oils with names you don't recognize or can't pronounce
All fats heated to very high temperatures in processing or frying
*Coconut Oil is by far the best. It is also the only oil that can withstand high temperatures when heated and will not change its composition.

On Eggs

Eggs have the highest quality protein found in any food and are packed full of vitamins, minerals, and amino acids. This is why I ate them everyday—*raw*.

Moreover, eggs are especially good at building muscle and contain 8 essential amino acids in the proportion regarded as the most bio available to the human body.

Here are a few more reasons to consider raw eggs in your diet—and to not leave out the yolks:

> Eggs do not raise cholesterol (contrary to popular belief)
> Egg yolks contain naturally occurring vitamin D
> Egg yolks contain choline
> Egg yolks contain vitamin A
> Egg yolks contain vitamin E
> Egg yolks contain lutein, which protects eyesight
> Eggshell membrane is a natural source of glucosamine, chondroitin, collagen, and hyaluronic acid.

Eggshell membrane contains the same substances as human joints, which means it's good for arthritis sufferers.

So, unless you have an egg allergy, raw eggs are highly recommended on my list. Moreover, if you are worried about salmonella, research shows the odds of contracting that are 1 in 20,000. (If that does happen, then probiotics or activated charcoal would be the protocol.) Please see www.food-healing.com for more information; however, consult your physician to find out whether eggs are right for you.

Raw Egg Smoothie Recipe

2-3 organic raw eggs
1 ½ cups purified water
¼ tablespoon organic unsalted butter
5 ½ tablespoons coconut oil (in liquid state)
¼ teaspoon nutmeg
¼ teaspoon cinnamon
Pinch of stevia
Pinch of spirulina, if desired
Pinch of chlorella, if desired

Mix lightly in blender on medium speed. Pour into a large glass or mug, and enjoy!

Chapter 6

What Can I Eat, and Is it Going To Taste Good?

Ultimately, yes. It's going to taste delicious.

Well, eventually it will. Your taste buds are probably accustomed to the sweet stuff, but remember, the sweet stuff got you into trouble in the first place, in excessive amounts and over time.

So the idea, or protocol, now is to change. As the old saying goes, if you want something different, then do things differently. Yes, taste was an issue, but for now my main objective was to get well—and stay well.

That was the promise I made to both Dr's, but even more to myself. That meant eating a lot of the green stuff. Yep, vegetables, mostly the green ones, but not all the time. The good news is it is going to taste okay at first, then progressively better, then absolutely delicious over time. That time frame varies, depending on the individual.

Here's the good, the bad and the ugly. Most of us eat for taste, not nutrition—but who says nutritious food's got to taste bad? Hippocrates, the ancient Greek physician, famously said, "Let food be thy medicine and medicine be thy food."

I began to study nutrition and learned that the blood needs to be alkaline, approximately 7.4 pH, known as homeostasis; less than that means it is more acidic. That acidic condition can cause us a lot of health problems. For that reason, we need to eat 75% alkaline-forming foods. The "green stuff," as I call it, is not only very nutritious but also alkalizing to the body. As weak as I was, I was prepared to jump into the pool feet first to take this unpopular plunge.

So, I prepared everything I ate—*everything*. I cooked every night when I came home from work and made sure there was enough for my lunch the next day. At the beginning of this process, I discovered that most adults with these health challenges have compromised immune systems. When a person's immune system is compromised, digestion is more difficult due to low enzyme production.

That being said, the food must be cooked (even lightly) to assist in breaking down the enzymes in the food for the body to be able to assimilate them better. So yes, I cooked most of my food. For breakfast I had the raw egg smoothie, which was the only raw food I had at that time; everything else was cooked.

An example of my lunch at that time was baked, skinless chicken that was hormone free and antibiotic free, with a side of cooked cabbage prepared with onion, garlic and coconut oil sauce. Sometimes I would have baked, wild-caught salmon or perch, with a side of zucchini and onions. On another day I might have a large bowl of cooked broccoli and cauliflower mix or just a stir-fried vegetable medley. I learned how to mix it up, and, yes, it was delicious.

The only other small challenge I had was that, at work, we had only a microwave oven. So I purchased a small toaster oven and, before lunchtime, I would reheat the meals I had previously prepared the night before. During my study and investigation, I had discovered that microwaving irradiates food. Radiation changes the molecular structure of the foods we eat. Why buy all this organic food and prepare it if you're going to zap it for two minutes in the microwave, destroy the nutrients, and turn your meal into what may be a harmful substance, even a carcinogen? The toaster oven was well worth the small investment.

My days and nights were very routine back then. I was never a person who liked much routine, but I had to do it to stay alive.

And I realized that routine is okay, and I even began to enjoy it. It allowed me to see things in a different light. It gave me an appreciation for my life and others, a gratitude to Source. I became more humble and compassionate. I had thought I was a compassionate person before my illness, but I now had a newfound humility and compassion I'd not known before.

Chapter 7

Changing Your Environment: Making Your Space a Healing Place Conducive to Wellness

I was really fortunate in that I was able to purchase a home shortly after my health challenges began. The market was down, and I was able to get a pretty good deal—not a great deal, but a really, really good one. The house was built about 3 years before I purchased it and looked almost new. The previous owners, unfortunately, had just lost it, and I felt bad for them and still wish them well.

The house, my new home, needed a little work, but I envisioned my healing taking place in it. I began to transform every room into a healing space.

I began by clearing out all the old stagnant and negative energy using purified water and affirmations. On a separate occasion, I used white sage in a "smudging" ceremony. Sage is an herb used for centuries to purify and cleanse.

I also repaired everything in my new home to like-new and working condition, including the light fixtures, furnace, and fireplace. I had the entire carpet shampooed and the hardwood floors polished. Then, I painted the entire home an uplifting, Caribbean color. Color, I discovered, affects your mood, so I chose Caribbean Coral. It was lively and bright. It spoke life to me.

The kitchen was a very important room to organize, and to start, I knew I had to have pure water. I began buying high-pH alkaline water and spring water. I would drink the high-pH water and use the spring water to make tea and to cook and prepare meals with. It was expensive at first, but I'm glad I did it. Eventually I purchased a water filter for the sink and began filling up jugs at the local food co-op and health food store. This saved me lots of money and was vastly more convenient.

Most of my shopping was also done at the local health food store. All the while, I still ate very little meat, mostly organic (cage-free, hormone-free, antibiotic-free) chicken and wild-caught fish.

And as I shopped, I observed how organized the store was. I thought, Why duplicate the wheel? Just take the same basic principle, adapt it and set up your kitchen that way. I saw how they had their herbs in glass jars with alphabetized labels on them, so I purchased glass jars, herbs and labels and went home to set up my pantry the same way.

I threw away any items in the refrigerator and pantry that I used to call "food," some with ingredients I could not pronounce, and replaced practically everything. I made sure that just about everything was an organic vegetable, with a few non-citrus fruits (except for lemons) and herbs. No sugar, none at all.

When I was done, my kitchen looked like the wellness section of a health food store.

This is when I really first began my food-based healing.

Chapter 8

Food Is Everything You Think: Change Your Thinking and Change Your World

Food is not just a physical thing. Everything you take in can feed your body, mind, and spirit. Even negative images and energy can have detrimental effects on your healing.

I was so desperate to heal that I stopped watching most TV programs. I watched only a few select shows, the ones that made me laugh, for about an hour a day. Laughter, I discovered, is very therapeutic and healing. When you laugh you live in the Now, not thinking about past tragedy or future anticipation. No anxiety, just funny *now* stuff—good, clean, and funny.

I realized that everything, *everything* we do can either help or hurt us: every word we speak, every sound we hear—everything.

Moreover, every thought we think can and does affect us. As my mother always says, "Think happy thoughts." She has keen mother-wit, as we called it, and although she may not have fully realized it on a conscious level, subconsciously she gave me the recipe to heal myself. Dr. Mark Armstrong, of the Ahimki Center for Wholeness, says, "As a woman thinketh, so is she," and "Where the mind goes, energy flows."

I knew I needed to make everything count in a positive way. I began to learn that even though there are many foods that can help you heal, some foods are even more beneficial than others. Highly alkalizing foods, such as asparagus, are more beneficial than green beans.

So I compared kale, broccoli, greens, spinach, collards, zucchini, peas, and a lot of the other green leafies. I ate them all, but I tried to eat more of the more alkaline ones. Learning and understanding this was huge in my healing. I realized that I had a choice, when I was shopping, that variety is good, but that when I had a choice, I would make the better choice for my healing.

Chapter 9

Excuses, Attachments, and Cheeta Willies: Organic Foods Cost Too Much

When I began shopping for food, I knew it had to be pure, or at least as pure as I could get it. And that meant organic produce, produce high in vitamins and other nutrients, and without chemicals and pesticides sprayed all over them. Vegetables—I didn't eat any fruit because of its high sugar content—in their most natural state.

Buying produce like this meant that it had to be purchased and eaten quickly. In order to do this, I began shopping every three days. Because organic food does cost a little more, this endeavor became quite costly and time consuming. I not only had a full time job, which was exhausting and depleting my energy, but now I had a health challenge that was going deep into my pockets and taking up more time in the kitchen than I had planned.

As mentioned previously, when I discovered the detrimental effects of microwave ovens, I stopped using them. This meant spending more time in the kitchen for food preparation.

But I could not, would not, and do not make excuses for any of it. I could not be attached to the money or the time that I used to have. The Cheeta Willies (my term for attachments) began to surface, and I had to not allow them to stay in my head. The best medicine I used was to laugh it off. At least, that's what I did when I wasn't dozing off from exhaustion.

As far as attachments go, foods can be addicting. For me it was, 'But I like my potatoes.' I call it the *But I Like My* syndrome. Most of us have foods we're partial to, and mine was potatoes. What kind of potatoes? Fried potatoes, baked potatoes, mashed potatoes, red potatoes, white potatoes, you name it. If it was made of potatoes, I wanted it—and I also had to give it up.

To be honest, once a month I would indulge in a side order of potatoes. I stress the term, *side order*. But when I did that, they were real organic potatoes that the body knew how to absorb. Even so, I always chased it down with several tablespoons of coconut oil in order to give the good, friendly bacteria a chance to proliferate and not feed the bad stuff with the carbs in the potatoes.

Okay, yeah, I know I still cheated. I admit it. But mentally, I feel you have to allow an indulgence every now and then. I had the equivalent of a small cup of real potatoes once a month with coconut oil and, if I could, depending on where I was, I added onion, garlic or both to help with the good stuff as well.

I'm not advocating or condoning cheating. By all means, if you can never cheat and stay on a healthy diet 100% of the time, then of course that's best. My recommendation is that if you do cheat, it's better to do it with an organic food in a small quantity. Now do what you will with that information, but don't blame me if things don't go well because you're eating potatoes or the like everyday with coconut oil. Be careful. Food can be addicting.

If that's not challenging enough, sometimes other Cheeta Willies can try to interfere with your healing. A Cheeta Willy can also be defined as just something you can't put your finger on. It is a conflicting energy, a negativity, an entity that appears to not want you to succeed. It could be conscious or subconscious thinking, perhaps, that we can get more benefit from being ill than we can from being well. It could be, perhaps, sympathy from another, compassion, attention (like a child who has his parents' attention when he is sick) or even a disability check. This is why it is paramount that, if you want to heal from your affliction, everything inside and out, in, around, and through you, must all vibrate wellness. No mixed messages anywhere for Cheeta Willies to attack.

And if one comes up, laugh at it.

Chapter 10

Ahimki Blessing: Vibrations of Wellness

During my healing journey, I flew to my hometown, several states away two to three times a month and did IV infusions with Dr. T and IV infusions with Dr. Richardson in Atlanta. The visits were two days each, so, initially, I was getting four days of intense healing every month. I combined these boosts of healing energy with my diet, vitamin supplements, sea salt minerals, coffee enemas, detox baths, dry skin brushing, laughter and anything else I could think of. (See the Appendix regarding these modalities.)

I was tired of my journey of illness and began to consider other possible options in Atlanta. And then, during one of my organic shopping trips, I met an angel.

I call him that, but his name is Atun. I was looking for herbs in the bulk herb department that might possibly assist in my healing. He asked me if I needed some help finding things, and he was amazingly knowledgeable and had such a warm, generous spirit.

After we chatted for a bit, I thanked him, with herbs in hand, and he told me that he wanted to become a naturopath someday and take Dr. Mark's course. He does energy healing among other things.

Who? I asked. He told me that Dr. Mark Armstrong was a naturopath there in Georgia, and he was "bad." Bad, as in good? I asked him.

Yep. Spirit had answered my request to step up my healing once more. This was a huge step—no, a leap, to find another naturopath that does energy work in between my visits out of state. I got the information from my new friend Atun, and I made an appointment with Dr. Mark, as he calls himself, at the Ahimki Center For Wholeness.

My first appointment was in a week, and I was excited. When I entered, Dr. Mark greeted me. He greets all of his clients (and believes there are no "patients") using the word "beloved." "Greetings, Beloved," he said. The words flowed not only from his mouth, but also with his vibration. I felt welcome at Ahimki. I began several different treatments there, but my favorite was Ondamed.

The Ondamed frequency machine is like the Bach Flower Remedies on steroids. The Bach Flower Remedies are vibrational tinctures developed by Dr. Edward Bach in the 1930s. Dr. Bach captured the vibrations of flower blossoms to heal the emotions that are the underlying cause of illness, then bottled the tinctures to be ingested several drops at a time. Bach believed that most illness is caused on the emotional level before it manifests physically, and these tinctures can help to heal you of many ailments or afflictions.

Dr. Mark has the Ondamed, a machine that does the same thing. The machine has three parts: a belt, a brace, and the machine itself, which looks like a computer. I was first assessed by Dr. Mark, and then, after placing the belt on, was assessed by the machine. The assessment tells you what disturbances you have in the body. Then the machine is programmed to eradicate those disturbances through frequencies designed for each client. Now I had another wonderful healing modality to help with my healing and well-being. I began to go to Dr. Mark at Ahimki twice a month. These visits were in addition to, and in between, both Dr. Richardson's and Dr T's.

Although feeling drained at times, I was desperate and determined to heal. My journeys back and forth from the two MD's and Dr. Mark ND in Atlanta, and my full-time/overtime job, were exhausting, but I felt I had little choice. I had to work the overtime in order to afford it all because none of my visits were covered by insurance. However, I needed to get well at all costs, because being healthy is less costly than funeral expenses, and I decided I wanted to be here.

Many days and nights of unpredictable reactions ensued. Sometimes at night after Ondamed, I felt jittery. Now, I know it was my physical vibration being changed back into wellness, but then, it wasn't easy. My body was changing, but I was not always sure what it would do and when.

I was in such a depleted state that I felt very fatigued most of the time. When I had treatments, I felt fatigued, and when I didn't have treatments, I felt fatigued. I wondered at times whether what I was doing was really working, but then something deep inside me, a very small voice, said, Yes, just keep going.

⋆

So I did. I continued the uphill climb, whether I ran or walked or crawled up there, because I was determined. I knew that I would not, I could not, return to the maze of doctors who said there was nothing wrong with me, that it was all in my head. No way was I going back there. I decided that I was going to forge ahead no matter what.

Chapter 11

Pushing Through The Pain: My Departure from Work and a Higher Calling

With more symptoms eventually surfacing, rectal pain, inflammation, chest pain and burning, I took refuge in every ounce of physical, mental emotional and spiritual wellness.

But it was still slow. Extremely slow. After all, I did not get sick overnight. And as much as I wanted to, I would not and did not get well overnight.

It was quite difficult to heal on this journey while working everyday. I performed on the job while feeling extremely fatigued. Then I would collapse at home after work, and then be back up again the next day for my high-stress job.

I prayed for relief. I prayed for salvation. I prayed for deliverance. And finally, God, Spirit, The Ultimate One, granted me a way out.

The company I worked for offered me a severance/early retirement package that was actually pretty good. Not great, but certainly not bad, especially in a tough economy. I had just barely made the cutoff, with 21 years of service.

My prayers had been answered. I accepted the package with great delight. This was my chance, my opportunity to depart with respect, dignity and grace—and, ultimately, to heal fulltime. It took five more months before I was actually released, and it seemed like the longest five months of my life. I was suffering immensely. In fact, twice during that time I had so much physical distress and anxiety I went to see two separate doctors on two separate occasions to request a sick note. During my last thirty days I even incurred a back injury that placed me on light duty (although there was

★

really no such thing on my job). One doctor wrote me out for an entire week, that's how bad my symptoms were.

My last day could not come soon enough. When it did, my manager said, "Well, thank you soooo much, not only for tonight, but for all the years." He then gave me a hug and said, "If you change your mind, you can still come in tomorrow."

I gave him a little smile and said, "Thanks, but I have a higher calling." I had made the decision that I wanted to become a naturopathic physician in order to help others so they would not have to go through what I had gone through to be healed. I was getting better, but I promised the Ultimate One that I would help others. I chose to answer the call.

Chapter 12

Receiving the Dao, and Finally Seeing "The Way"

It was such a relief not having to get up out of bed and go to work. Since I was exhausted most of the time anyway, I slept in later than usual. Most days I just attempted to feel my legs in this new life of unemployment and uncertainty. I had lived on a lot less money before, so I knew what it would be like. And here I was again, with enough funds (if I budgeted right) to last me about a year. It would be a limited treatment year, but I knew that even with fewer treatments I would feel better without the stress of working everyday.

So, I continued to feel my way, researching online, purchasing books, going to the library and networking as much as I could. I was still exhausted during the process; I'd fall asleep while reading, or be nauseated on many occasions and jittery at home, hoping all of this would work.

My regime consisted of IV therapy in two states, chiropractic adjustments and acupuncture, and vitamin and mineral supplements. I also returned to Atlanta to see Dr. Mark and to be hooked up to the Ondamed machine. This was still combined with the all-important high protein, low carb diet of mostly green leafies. I kept modifying and adjusting the diet to fit my lifestyle, but now I could make it better since my time was now my own.

Meanwhile, I was free—free, but exhausted. Approximately one month later, while hooked up to Ondamed, Dr. Mark said to me, "Greetings, Beloved. I'm leaving for Temple early today. Are you familiar with Dao?"

"Huh?" I responded, with my eyes barely open while sitting in the treatment chair.

He said, "Yes, the Dao. I go to the Dao Temple and I'd like to invite you to receive the Dao."

I asked him what it was. He replied, "Dao is The Way." He left the room and returned with a sheet of paper for me. It said the Dao can assist you in revealing your true heart. It leads to self-realization and helps you to understand the Truth of Life.

My first impression was that it sounded great. Moreover, if Dr. Mark was involved and recommended it, then I should strongly consider it. The only reservation I had was that I did not want to get involved in another religion. I had been involved with so many religions in my life that I just wanted to have my personal relationship with God, The Ultimate One, without the judgments of others. Just as I was thinking that, Dr. Mark said, "It's not a religion," as if reading my mind.

So, I found myself in my car on the way to the Dao Temple, thirty-seven days after leaving corporate America. Not having been there before, naturally I got lost—I mean, really lost.

The temple was about an hour's drive from my home outside Atlanta. I called the number on the paper Dr. Mark had given me and got directions from three separate people and still could not find the temple. I'd almost given up when a small voice inside me said, "Keep going." This voice was usually correct, but it was still frustrating at times because I knew I should listen even though it made me feel uncomfortable.

I arrived and walked in almost two hours late. I wanted to apologize, to tell someone that at least I knew where they were now and would be there on time for the next ceremony, but as I entered, I felt a genuine rush of love. The feeling enveloped me completely, and before me stood a gentle, loving spirit with a name badge that read "Darla." The loving spirit had a smiling face and a warm voice that said, "Welcome. You must be Charise, and you are right on time." She bowed and I sort of bowed back. She asked me to remove my shoes, symbolic of leaving the outside, outside. She bowed again and handed me a warm, clean, wet cloth and asked me to finish the process by cleaning my hands. I followed her instructions, and she led me into the temple.

My experience inside the Dao temple is a sacred one, an experience like no other. I always knew there existed a place on earth like this, pure, true, serene and protected. Yes, the Dao is not a religion. I love going to the Temple anytime I want and always feel welcome, enveloped in love. For a place that is not a religion, it draws people from every walk of life: rich, poor, black, white, Asian, Native American, everyone. Those who have affinity receive the Dao. *Wow.*

Thank you, Dr. Mark, for the invitation. I am forever humbly grateful to you and for having the affinity. I am grateful for Dao, God and Buddha for leading me to the place in my heart that I always knew was made of love, peace and everlasting joy.

Oh, and thank you to the small, tiny voice inside me that has always been right, saying, "Keep going."

Chapter 13

The Accident: Using My Gifts

Approximately two months after receiving the Dao I started taking a Tai Chi class. My energy was still low, but I had heard that Tai Chi might help.

At that first class, I observed the other students. It looked simple enough, so I began to try to emulate their movements. Then after about five minutes, I wanted some water. The instructor said, "Okay, it's your first day, go get some. After today, no more new student and no more water." I muttered a little under my breath and began the set again. It was difficult.

I returned the next week to continue and struggled through. I was embarrassed, but determined to get through each set, week after week.

Then something began to happen: my body began to change, I mean noticeably change. It felt stronger, from the inside. I really had incentive to continue going to each and every class. Until one day on my way to class I was driving on the interstate on my way to pick up a friend. At the exit, another vehicle spead passed me and cut me off and stopped short. Our vehicles made contact. The airbag deployed which fractured my wrist. After the impact I rememered my DAO treasures to be used in an emergency. As I rememered them, an individual appeared and assisted me until an ambulence came to take me to the hospital. I was blessed to have received DAO because it can help you in any urgent situation.

While in the ambulance, I was able to contact Sifu Armstrong (Master Armstrong) my Tai Chi Instructor. I explained to him that I would not be in class due to a major accident and that I was in an ambulance. He immediately asked about injuries, and when I said I had chest pain and a broken arm, he immediately said, "I will begin to heal you now. Just think about your arm and chest, okay?" I was crying profusely, but I said okay. I was unsure of what he was doing, but at that point I would accept any help. And miraculously, my arm felt different, as if the blood was moving.

From the ambulance I was able to notify my mother and sister, as well as two friends here in Georgia. My sister said, "I'm going to send you some Reiki, Sis. You're gonna be all right." That was my first experience with distant healing, and I knew that it was helping.

At the hospital, the doctors and nurses took six X-rays (that I objected to, but I had to comply because they would not stitch me up unless I did). Since I was a little uncooperative, to say the least, they shot me up with Morphine five times to calm me down. The two friends I had called from the ambulance, Tammy and Ralph, came into the room shortly afterward. They both took control, and really helped to settle me down. They talked to the doctors and nurses for me and with me. What a harrowing experience.

Chapter 14

Returning to Tai Chi

Although it had only been three days, my Tai Chi Instructor, Sifu Armstrong, whom I fondly call Sifu, urged me to get to him. Perplexed, I listened to that small inner voice again and complied.

When I entered the class, my classmates were very concerned and gave me hugs as they welcomed me back. Sifu (Master-Teacher) asked me to sit down. When I did, he looked me in the eye and said, "I'd like to take a look at your arm."

I showed him my arm, in the soft cast they'd put on me three days ago in the hospital.

"No, no," he said. "We gotta take that off." He sat down next to me and began unraveling the neatly wrapped surgical tape and splint. As he did, tears ran down my face, the silent ones that come from that deep, dark place of unforgiveness. I was unforgiving towards myself for making a mistake.

Sifu Armstrong immediately started breaking up the energy, sending it back to the earth from which it had come. My arm lay there limp, dark and lifeless as Sifu began to work on me with his partner and assistant, L'Inda. As I watched them work, the class stopped practicing and came over to watch as well. Sifu and L'Inda together moved Chi in my body to heal my arm and hand. They used sound as well, special compresses, snake oil, and a little moxibustion to aid in the healing.

After about forty minutes, he said, "Okay, get up and train."

I really wanted to laugh at that point. I mean, really hard and really loud. But I said, "You gotta be kidding me, right?" I looked at him and he looked at me. I turned to look at my classmates for some possible assistance.

They all looked down at the floor, moved away from us and returned to their previous positions to train again.

Sifu looked at them, then he looked at me and pointed to them, saying, "Join them." At this point, I had absolutely nothing on my arm—no splint, no tape, no cast, no nothing. He said, "Well, you can put a half sock on it if it makes you feel better, but it's best to let it be. The bones are already starting to heal so you don't need anything on it." I was thinking, Now wait a minute. My arm is broken in three places: at the wrist, behind the wrist, and on the arm itself. But the little small voice in my head said, "Get up. Join your class." So I slowly arose and did what my Sifu said. (You gotta do what your Sifu says!.)

As I began to raise my hands in the first move, my arm began to buckle. When I cried out in pain, Sifu said, "Don't think about it, just do it. You know it. You can do it."

So, I did it again and it worked. It worked like I'd never broken it. But when I would think about it, my arm would buckle and throb in pain again. My heart was also throbbing and beating faster than usual, as if someone had punched me in the chest. After about ten minutes, I sat down. Sifu said, "Great. Now it's time to meditate." After meditation, we were released to go home.

Sifu said, "I'll see you in a couple of days to work on you again. Whatever you do, I don't recommend you having a hard cast put on, it makes your arm atrophy."

"All right," I said, leaving as quickly as I could. I was so glad to get out of there and return home to rest.

But I put the splint on that night to sleep.

For the next two weeks, I listened to and did everything my Sifu said, and in no time at all, my left, broken arm looked and felt almost like my right, healthy arm. Percentage-wise, as I am writing this, it's about 92% and still improving. By and large, of course, I continued to train.

Chapter 15

Tai Chi For Real: Getting My Mojo Back

I mentioned previously that it was the Dao that saved my life. However, Tai Chi also healed me. It is important for me to stress what Tai Chi has done for me.

Before taking Tai Chi, I was a basket case. I was on the candida diet, weak, frustrated, depressed, nauseated, and I weighed 100 pounds soaking wet.

I constantly thought about my illness. It was literally always on my mind. Unknowingly, I identified myself with it. After all, it was my story—and my life and my health meant everything to me. It was superseded only by my relationship with God, The Ultimate One. I could not understand why God would allow this to happen to me. What was all of this for? What purpose could this serve? I identified with Jesus, who said, "God, why hast thou forsaken me?" I was ready and willing to try anything (well almost anything) to get well.

I'd heard about Tai Chi from my mother and sister, who both raved about it. So, I sought out a Tai Chi master in Atlanta and began taking his class. At that time, I didn't know what it truly was. I didn't even understand what I was doing at first, but I went and started doing the movements. However, I knew from that little, soft voice, that sometimes understanding comes later.

As time went on, something inside rang true and authentic for me. "Just keep going," my voice said, the same message I was getting a lot lately. After the accident I felt very discouraged, as if I had to start all over again. The first time had been hard enough, but beginning again seemed next to impossible.

Tears would well up in my eyes on many occasions. I didn't know why or what I was doing, but I would keep going. Even though I hardly ever practiced the moves at home, I would always go to class three times a week. I felt frustrated by my inability to do the movements at times, but exhilarated when I was able to accomplish them. As I kept attending the class, I understood more and more.

An epiphany for me happened one day when I started to realize that when I was doing the movements, I was not thinking about the illness or other problems in my life. I realized that the illness was not *mine*. The problems were not *mine*. It was if they did not exist. The illness did not exist because I did not exist, at least in this form. I was only using this form to accomplish what needed to be accomplished. So, the question became, "Where is Charise?" And the answer was, "Here and nowhere." So, if I am nowhere, then where is the illness? It is nowhere.

Wow. The principles that I was learning are not just physical, but universal. I was learning to blend and to not compete. When your body does it, your mind does it as well because it is one and the same. Body, Mind, Spirit—the same. Everything and everyone is you and there is no separateness, no competition, no struggle, flowing with nature, being unselfish, becoming unattached to everything, including illness and health.

Chapter 16

The Sun (Ra): Standing and Sitting in the Light

The Sun is such an amazing healing energy that I dedicate this chapter to my intimate friend, Ra.

I discovered that, contrary to what the media have been telling us, to stay out of the sun, it is the greatest healing energy there is. Father Sun and Mother Earth. I have so much love and respect for you both.

My healing journey led me directly to the Sun. First I discovered that each of us is made up of about seventy-two trillion cells, and that most causes of illness are from cell degeneration. Then, I discovered that each cell can be regenerated by the sun. So I asked myself, how do you regenerate the cells by the sun? The answer? By getting in the Sun, a lot of Sun, with sunlight on every part of your skin possible. Please see this link by Dr. Bernarr, DC. DD. www.healself.org.

Unfortunately, in this society, we can't walk around naked to achieve sunlight exposure everywhere on the body. However, I could sit outside on my front porch with a bikini on. So, that's what I did. Every morning when Ra began to appear, I greeted him in all his glory and in all my glory. Fortunately, there was not a lot of people-traffic outside my porch in the courtyard, except for the dog walkers and an occasional neighbor walking out the door in disbelief. But I needed to heal, so naked in the Sun (well, almost naked) I went.

Just taking this one loving, healing energy into my body everyday and with every opportunity did wondrous, amazing things for me. Despite the increased heart rate and rashes that occurred while the Sun pulled out the toxins, I began to feel a much greater sense of overall well-being.

First, I would ask Ra's permission to heal my body mind, spirit, and every aspect of my being. Once permission was granted, my healing was on. Ra would envelope me in his Love, and it is a feeling unlike any other. Being in the open air and feeling the Sunlight on your skin is amazingly awesome.

Then I discovered Sun-gazing. This is the process of looking at the Sun at sunrise or sunset in sequential seconds, starting at a couple of seconds and building up everyday until you get to about 60 seconds. This process takes months and months to achieve. It has to be done following instructions exactly, so as not to do damage to your eyes. Do it only if you already know how or are under the supervision of a master. When I added a little Sun-gazing to my healing practice, I started to heal in leaps and bounds.

I experienced standing barefoot on Mother Earth while bringing up electromagnetic energy and pulling down healing rays from Father Sun, as love exemplified.

Love is always here. Seize it, embrace it, look for it, live it, be it. We are part of everything and everything is a part of us. Love is the highest vibration in the universe.

Ra and Earth: I love, love, love you both.

Chapter 17

Good Night: Catching some Zzzzzzz's.

As the day would wind down, so would I.

I began to go to bed earlier and earlier. While I was working at my job, I had never gone to bed before 1:30 or 2:00 a.m. But my newfound discoveries had led me to the healing aspects of sleep—not only getting enough sleep, but the proper times for sleep. By living in accordance with the circadian cycle of the Earth, where one sleeps during darkness and rises or awakens during daylight, one is living healing personified. During the day the sun helps the body create serotonin. At night, when the body is at rest, it releases melatonin, which aids in healing. It is released into the cells and organs during that time. The sun helps to create this magnificent healing ability.

It is presumed that, during certain parts of the night, healing takes place at particular, appointed times. I discovered that our bodies repair their organs at night, and we have our own built-in maintenance times:

Blood Vessels & Arteries	9p.m.-11p.m.
Gallbladder	11p.m.-1a.m.
Liver	1a.m.-3a.m.
Lungs	3a.m.-5a.m.
Large Intestine	5a.m.-7a.m.
Stomach	7a.m.-9a.m.
Spleen	9a.m.-11a.m.
Heart	11a.m.-1p.m.

Small Intestines	1p.m.-3p.m.
Bladder	3p.m.-5p.m.
Kidneys	5p.m.-7p.m.
Pancreas	7p.m.-9p.m.

These times are for the repair and maximum performance of specific organs during each day. This is called the circadian rhythm cycle of one day, or the body clock.

So, I began to retire to bed earlier and earlier. Sometimes it's still a challenge, but I now know that my body cannot heal properly if it is deprived of sleep.

Chapter 18

Tweaking The Program

What to do now, I wondered.

I was spending time in the sun, but I still needed more healing.

I was spending a small fortune on treatments, supplements and organic food. Although weak, I was actually feeling better. Between research, visits to the naturopaths, grocery shopping every couple of days for fresh produce, Tai Chi three days a week, and taking the time to prepare meals, I had little time for anything else. All these things, of course, took up every ounce of strength and every free minute of every day. Wasn't there anything, and I mean *anything*, that could enhance or speed up my progress even more?

So, everyday during my research, I continued to look for new healing modalities, exercises, herbs, products, or ways of thinking that might help. When I found something, I thought about it, considered adding it, and often did, as long as my body was ready for it and it was not harmful. I incorporated things into my already busy schedule and put together my own program.

I became my own experiment. I tried things out as if this body were separate from me, almost like a science project. I constantly stepped out of my body to ask it questions, like, "Do you want more raw eggs? "Do you want protein shakes?" "How about raw food?"

And my body would answer me by way of kinesiology, which is a form of muscle testing. This is how it is done: While standing straight, I'd ask my body a question while placing my hands on my chest. If my body moved forward while standing still, it meant my body was accepting of the food or modality. If it moved slightly back, then that meant not to eat it or try it. Since the body is designed to heal itself, it can always tell you what it wants. Since everything is energy, I was beginning to learn how to use it.

I began adding things in and taking things out according to what my body wanted. Here is a list of things that I ultimately tried and did on various occasions, according to the answers my body gave me:

Amalgam filling removal
Acupuncture
Acupressure
Bach Flower Remedies
Baking soda enemas
Being happy
Being around health-conscious people
Being around higher vibration people
Chiropractic adjustments
Coffee enemas
Colon hydrotherapy
Crystals
Detox baths
Detox kits and cleanses
Diode plates
Doing affirmations
Doing mantras
Dry skin brushing
EFT
Eliminating microwaves
Frequency balancing
Getting rid of toxic substances in the home
Going braless (freeing up the lymphatic system)
Green superfoods
Herbs
High pH water
Humidifier/air cleaner
Laughing
Massage and lymphatic massage
Meditation
Ondamed
Orgons
Oxygen

⭐

Prayer
Qi Gong
Reiki
Rebounding
Rosaflora Flower Essences
Saunas
Sleeping during the appropriate times
SRS (Dr. Mark Armstrong's program)
Sun-gazing at sunrise and sunset
Sunlight (on every part of skin)
Tai Chi
Thumping the thymus
Wearing diodes
Wheatgrass
Yoga

I'm sure there may have been a few more. (I go into each one of these in the companion manual to this book)

I finally realized that I was my own Cavalry. No one was coming over the hill to save me, but with Heaven's Grace, I would save myself.

I discovered in a class at Ahimki, called Healing Hands of Light, that illness does not start in the body. Something precipitated it, usually a feeling. So I researched further and discovered Louise Hay's book, *You Can Heal Your Life*, and another book, *Feelings Buried Alive Never Die* by Karol K Truman, also the title of another Ahimki Class.

Conclusion? A major component of illness is housed in unforgiveness.

Chapter 19

Forgiving Everyone Means Forgiving Yourself

This whole journey allowed me to take a look at myself. I mean, really take a look inside—examining every aspect and fiber of my being.

Was there anyone whom I had not forgiven? And why? Or was it myself that I needed to forgive? I began to do this inventory and came up with a few folks. I had childhood friends, teachers, parents, siblings, children, co-workers, relatives and ex-husbands that could have all been on the list. I had always been a pretty forgiving person, but I had to admit, even to myself, that more forgiveness was in order.

During my meditations, I would often see the white light. The white light is pure, heavenly, perfect, serene, and bright. I began seeing the individuals who I felt had wronged me in the past in my meditations and would send them into the white light. One by one, they would go. This exercise transmuted the pain into love. It was like I was giving myself a forgiveness shot every time I meditated.

However, while going within, I discovered the worst demon of all: the wrongs that I had done to myself. I had not forgiven myself for the pain I had inflicted upon others, and equally upon myself, no matter how great or how small the harm. It was most important now that my meditations include, first and foremost, the forgiving of myself.

During the course of my life, I had participated in a few counseling sessions (mainly marital counseling). I'd never considered myself to be out of balance mentally or even emotionally. I was fortunate to grow up in a two-parent household with a lot of love, an emphasis on education and hard work. Of course, we had our problems, as no one in this life or on this planet can escape traumas, dramas, some sadness or hard times. However, meditation was, and is, the best therapy.

All of the answers that we seek are inside our own mind. All we have to do is sit still long enough, quiet our thoughts, listen to our heart and send love out to each and every person we have not forgiven. For each and every person is also us. We are they, and they are we. It is our reflection that we see when we look at them.

So, we sit cross-legged in the five-point star position, close our two outer eyes, breathe through the abdomen while envisioning the white light coming through our third eye (which is actually our first eye), and forgive. As we forgive everyone for everything and forgive ourselves for everything, we heal our bodies, minds, and spirits. Moreover, we attain the peace, joy, and love we desperately seek.

And the best part is, it does not cost anything except the time and right intention to do it.

Chapter 20

Pulling It All Together

I really started to feel as if I was living a brand new life. I had journeyed so far down the rabbit hole that I began to come out the other side. My whole body had changed, along with my disposition and my mind.

I am a whole new person, with greater life and vitality. Moreover, I am humbly grateful. I didn't realize that I had it in me. I'm careful to remember, though, that it has not been just me. I have received the grace without which nothing can be accomplished. I bow in humility when I see others recognizing the divine in each one.

My advice? Stay the course. I still stay the course. Food, real food, tastes fabulous now. My senses are even more keen. My taste buds are now heightened and I have no desire to go back to eating junk food—none. Food nourishes me, and I now actually have fuel to accomplish things without tiring. I feel liberated and free, realizing I have everything I need. I am following nature and living life the way it was and is intended to be lived. I'm not worrying about my next meal or shelter, like the birds and the bees and the flowers and trees. They are all here to teach us how to live.

I realize a lot of people have financial stresses, emotional traumas and physical limitations. However, we all have tools and examples in Nature to teach us and care for us. All we need to do is listen, watch, emulate and learn from her.

You have everything you need to vastly improve, if not heal, your life. Have faith and it can happen. It will happen. As Dr. Mark at Ahimki says, "Where the mind goes, energy flows." Since our minds are major transmitters and receivers, we can bring in and send out anything. You have to believe it and do it. If you want to heal, you truly can. Period.

Remember, the illness is not you. Never claim it. Claim health and vitality. Speak it into existence. When people ask, "How are you?" say, "I am well, thank you."

So, do the diet. Meditate, drink good water and get the sun while standing barefoot on the planet.

It is your choice—yours and only yours. Stay positive. When things seem overwhelming, remind yourself that others have healed themselves and you can too. The longest journey begins with the first step, putting one foot in front of the other. When it appears to be bleak, remember the saying, "How do you eat an elephant? One bite at a time."

Always keep it moving, for life is movement. Stagnation is death. You are worth it. Every nickel you spend on yourself is a wise investment. Your money is worthless to you if you are not around to spend it. The time you spend on yourself is valuable to you and can be valued more to others if you are healthy and here to share it with them.

This is your gift to yourself and your gift to humanity. Offer it freely, like the birds offer food to their young, and one day you will fly.

I'll see you up there beside me.

Chapter 21

Crossing The Finish Line: Your Investment in Yourself

What better investment can one make, than an investment in oneself? If you don't believe in you, how can you expect anyone else to?

If you want to be well, I mean truly want and desire to be well with every fiber of your being, then you have to vibrate that. Radiate it. Sing it. Feel it. Sleep it. Everything in your conscious mind and your subconscious mind has to radiate wellness. Even if it is only a small flicker of light right now, you have to consciously and subconsciously hold the space for it to be a brilliant, constant, non-ending, almost blinding Sun inside of you. It is everywhere and nowhere. It is you. Hold it in your mind everyday, for all the day, always. Constantly.

Everything in this universe, everything in the cosmos, bends toward you being well. You are not sick. The body may have a little health challenge, but you are not your illness. Don't view yourself as your body. You do, and always will, exist. Death only happens to the body, if you let it. (Another topic for later.) Cultivate you. Elevate you, the real you. The body will take care of the rest. It will heal itself.

Don't allow thoughts of anger or unforgiveness to fester. When you feel anger, change your thoughts and do it as quickly as possible. The longer you hold on to it the more it gets locked into your cellular memory and creates dis-ease. Really, most of our "stuff" is so really unimportant, or at least not as urgent as we allow it to be.

When you don't forgive, you bury two people: yourself, and the person you're not forgiving. Moreover, they've probably moved on with their life while you get sicker and sicker, holding on to your resentment. So, do yourself a favor and let it go. We all know the old saying, "Let go and let God." Well, whatever your belief system, no one gets away with anything.

Why? Scientifically, it's cause and effect, the Yin and Yang of life. So, if you don't want harm, then cause no harm. If you want love, then give love. Give what you want to get and it will return to you. Do not be concerned with outcome. Just do good deeds, help others, serve others, whether you think they deserve it or not. Are you really in a position to judge whether someone else is worthy? When the rain falls, or the sun shines, there is no discrimination. It shines and falls down upon the Earth to all creatures on the planet. So, be grateful, eternally grateful, that you do not have to ask or beg for your sustenance, that it is given from the heavens freely unto you. Be grateful. I am.

Your life was ordained. It has a purpose and a reason. You chose to be here. If you are sick, choose again. Choose to be well. *Choose.* Choose to stay here and be here again. Through your choices and by Heaven's Grace, you will not only survive, you will thrive.

I'm not saying it's easy, but it can be less difficult. If you make the choice, then you should honor it. You cheat no one but yourself if you don't. You hurt no one but yourself if you don't. Furthermore, if you receive the Grace to be healed, be grateful and humble. Remember to pay it forward. Help others to see the light. Always remember what it was like when you were in the dark and could not find your way. Learn the lessons on your journey. Unlock your own gates to wellness. Only you have the key. Your body will respond to your Authentic Self.

Summing it Up

Everything is energy, vibrating at different speeds. That means that we are a part of everything and everything is a part of us.

So, how does one manage to vibrate sickness instead of health? Or, a better question, how can one vibrate health—no, *vibrant* health, instead of sickness?

If the mind is in everything and everything is in the mind, then potential sickness and vibrant health exist there. If the mind is the major transmitter of everything, then why not emit and transmit what you desire?

Okay, let's rewind the tape. If this is true, then an appropriate question to ask ourselves might be, "What was I thinking before I got sick?" The process would be to regress for just a moment, think about what we were thinking before we became ill.

That's exactly what I did. Then, I immediately sent it love. It's like erasing a tape and recording over it, imprinting a whole new frequency upon your cells. It is literally reprogramming yourself. Where there was once pain, there is now Love. The frequency of love is the highest vibration that there is.

So, I suggest to you that you don't think about your illness—think about wellness. Think about how you are Vibrantly Healthy Now. See yourself in your mind's eye as healthy, as doing the activities that you want to do. Envision it, and feel it. I know that, at times, it may appear to be difficult, but it is necessary and vital to your healing.

It will never happen unless you do it. Let me say it again: Healing will never happen unless you do it. If it seems too difficult, try these things: Make a point to read, think or watch something that is uplifting or funny. Do not live in or occupy a space of illness. Grow the part of you that is healthy, until vibrant health is abundant and running rampant throughout your being.

⭐

    Laughing is important. When you laugh, you exist in the Now. A lot of our illness comes from anguish about the past or anticipation or fear of the future. Well, all any of us has is Now, and that Now is experienced when you laugh. So, when you find something to be funny, laugh as loud and as long as you can. You'll be surprised at what it will do for your body, let alone your mind and your spirit.

Divine Love
And
Eternal Light.
Chi

Awaken Your Healing
Power Now.

Tai Chi/Qi Gong Update

Well, It's been a little over a year as of this writing since I began my Tai Chi Qi Gong practice. I can truly say that I have much greater inner peace, one which I have never experienced before. I've also gained about 25 much-needed pounds consisting mostly of firm muscle mass. My body has more inner and outer strength, definition, vitality and flexibility.

I also have a profound settled-ness inside that I have not known before. I developed more inner strength, love, compassion, joy and peace, feeling more grounded and connected to not only myself but to nature, the planet, the heavens and to all things.

Yes, Tai Chi improves your physical body, bending and stretching, turning the waist, massaging the organs. But the overall benefit is so much more. It is an expression of how life should be lived. You won't understand that, unless you do it, and it happens immediately, yet subtly.

Tai Chi will always be there, even when no one or nothing else is. It will never fail you or become fickle or change. It's the yin and yang of life. If you want to be well, I recommend doing Tai Chi.

I realize I've only scratched the surface. I still struggle and sweat through the movements most days. However, when I do I give the Tai Chi Smile. I know I am still yet a babe in the practice, but at least now I've been born.

Thank you, Sifu Armstrong, and L'Inda.

I continue to train.

Glossary

Acupressure—A form of therapy similar to acupuncture that uses manual pressure rather than needles on acupuncture sites on the body

Acupuncture—An ancient method of therapy and pain relief that involves puncturing specific sites of the body with needles

Affirmation—A positive statement that asserts that a goal the speaker or thinker wishes to achieve is already happening

AHIMKI—Ahimki Center For Wholeness located in Roswell Georgia offers a variety of modalities to help restore balance and harmony to body, mind and spirit. Naturopathic Educational Program Founder and Director Dr. Mark Armstrong.

Amalgam Filling—A substance used as filling for tooth cavities, consisting of a paste of powdered mercury, silver, and tin that quickly hardens

Atlanta Clinic of Preventative Medicine—Dr. William Richardson MD ND www.acpm.net

Bach Flower Remedies—A healing system that uses the vibrational essences of 37 wildflowers for physical, emotional, mental and spiritual healing developed in the 1930's by British physician, Dr. Edward Bach

Baking Soda Enema—The insertion of a liquid infusion containing baking soda into the bowels via the rectum as a treatment to cleanse the colon of waste

Chelation Therapy—To treat with a chelating agent in order to remove toxic heavy metals, such as mercury and lead, from the bloodstream

Chiropractic Adjustment The manipulation and adjustment to re-align spinal vertebrae that have gotten out of alignment in order to reduce pain and inflammation

Coffee Enemas—The insertion of a liquid infusion containing coffee into the bowels via the rectum as a treatment to cleanse the colon of waste

Colon Hydrotherapy; Colon Irrigation—The gentle infusion of pure, warm water into the colon via the rectum to cleanse and heal the colon of accumulated waste

Crystals—Crystalline substances, usually minerals containing quartz, that have semi-conducting or piezoelectric properties that can affect the bio-electric system of the human body to promote balance and healing

DAO or Tao—A Chinese word meaning, "The Way". The object of spiritual practice is to become one with the Tao or to harmonize one's will with Nature

Dermatologist—A physician who specializes in diagnosing and treating problems and diseases of the skin

Detox Bath—A bath treatment to rid the body of toxic substances in which the water may contain mineral salts, essential oils and other essences of plants to facilitate the process

Digestive Enzyme—A complex protein produced in the digestive system that aids in the breaking down of foods to be assimilated and used by the body

Diodes—An electronic plate in which are imbedded two electrodes that convert alternating current to direct current.

Dry Skin Brushing—To use a bristle brush or loofa to brush the skin directionally towards the colon in order to circulate lymph fluids that carry waste to be eliminated from the body

EFT—A healing system that involves tapping various acupuncture meridian points to release the subconscious mind of deep, negative beliefs and feelings in order to free oneself from pain and negativity and come back into harmony

EP2 Stress Reducing Pendant—helps restore and protect the body from ongoing assault of abundance of electronic chaos. Ultimate cell phone and environmental chaos protection. www.ewater.com/ADWellness

Fasting—The act of abstaining from some or all food, drink, or both, for a period of time to allow the body to remove toxins, increase energy, restore health and gain spiritual clarity

Food Co-op—A market or store in which members buy their food cooperatively to promote buying from local food producers, to foster community, and to receive bulk pricing

Frequency Balancing—An energy healing technique in which chi energy is sent to the client using healing frequencies and other tools to reduce stress and eliminate imbalances and blockages within the human energy system

Grace—The infinite love, mercy, favor and goodwill shown to humankind by God/Goddess/All That Is/Creator/Great Spirit

Green Superfoods—Natural foods, usually in powder form, comprised of concentrated, easily digestible nutrients, such as disease-fighting fruits, vegetables, microalgae, probiotics, and sea vegetables, that can enhance health and increase energy

Gynecologist—A physician who specializa Physisicianes in the treatment of the female reproductive system

Happiness—To be in a state of spontaneous joy, love and gladness

Higher-Vibration Person—A person who feels positive, energized and optimistic; a person whose presence uplifts those around them

☆

Health-Conscious Person—A person who is concerned with the health of their body, takes responsibility to educate themselves about healthy options for their body, and attempts to follow a lifestyle of eating nutritious foods, exercise and fostering positive thoughts and feelings

Herbs—Low-growing aromatic plants used fresh or dried for seasoning in cooking, for their medicinal properties, or in perfumes. Sage and rosemary are herbs.

High PH Water (You're not sick you're dehydrated)—Alkaline water that may neutralize acid in the bloodstream, boost metabolism and help prevent disease and aging

Humidifier/Air Cleaner—A device or machine that removes particles and dust from the air and keeps the air moist inside an enclosed space

Hypnotherapy—The use of hypnosis in treating illness, for example, in dealing with physical pain or psychological problems

IV—Intravenous therapy used in administering fluids or medicines into the veins

Laughing—To laugh spontaneously at times of great fun and enjoyment; an action that helps reduce stress, boost the immune system and body's healing response

Kinesiology—a system of muscle testing that reveals and corrects musculoskeletal imbalances and identifies food sensitivities.

Light—A spiritual illumination that is a divine attribute or the embodiment of divine truth; the underlying essential composing element of space and the cosmos, of which visible light is a manifestation

Lymphatic System—A part of the body's circulatory system that is comprised by a network of vessels that carry clear fluid called lymph that filters blood and helps to fight infection

Lymphatic Massage—A technique used to encourage lymph flow in the body to reduce body toxins, waste and improve metabolism

MD—Medical Doctor

Mantra—A sacred word, chant, or sound that is repeated during meditation to facilitate spiritual power and transformation of consciousness

Massage Therapy—The manipulation of body tissues by stroking, kneading, and tapping to improve muscle tone, circulation, reduce muscle tension, stress, and to prevent disease and restore health

Meditation—The emptying of the mind of thoughts, or concentration of the mind on just one thing, in order to aid mental or spiritual development, contemplation, or relaxation

Microwave—A type of electromagnetic wave whose wavelength ranges from 1.0 mm to 30 cm, used in radar, to carry radio transmissions, and in cooking or heating devices—used in microwave ovens

Naturopath; Naturopathic Doctor (ND)—A physician licensed and trained in using natural methods and therapies to prevent or treat disease

Neurologist—A physician who specializes in the diagnosis and treatment of disorders affecting the nervous system

ONDAMED—a device or machine that uses vibrational energy to facilitate and support healing in the body

Ophthalmologist—A physician who specializes in eye and vision care

Organic Foods—Fruits, vegetables and grains that come from crops that are not sprayed with insecticides and are certified as organic by a national organization

RA, or **RE**—The midday sun of ancient Egypt

Oxygen Therapy—A type of medical treatment that uses oxygen to promote, speed up and sustain healing in the body

PCP—Primary Care Provider or a health care practitioner who sees people with common medical problems

POA Workshop—Power Of Awareness is a powerful program that assists one to discover and recover one's own magnificence. Founded and Directed by Laina Orlando at the Center For Awareness in Marietta Georgia. www.thePowerofAwareness.com

Prayer—A humble approach to God/Goddess/All That Is/Creator/Great Spirit in words, thoughts, petition, praise, devotion, worship, adoration or thanksgiving

Reiki—A treatment in holistic medicine in which Chi or Qi healing energy is channeled through the practitioner to the patient to enhance energy and reduce stress, pain, and fatigue

Rosaflora Flower Essences—A system of healing liquid tinctures made from the energetic imprints of more than 75 species and cultivated roses, which are used to facilitate spiritual healing and a shift to higher consciousness. www.rosaflora.net

SRS—Stress Reversal System which helps heal and clear pain on all levels. Physical, mental, emotional, ethercal, and astral. Originator and Founder Dr. Mark Armstrong. www.Ahimki.net

Sauna—A kind of therapeutic bath that involves a time in a hot, steamy room in order to cleanse the body

Supplements—Herbs, minerals or vitamins in pill or capsule form, usually taken by mouth to support the nutritional needs of the body that may not be acquired from foods

Tai Chi—A Chinese form of physical exercise characterized by a series of very slow and deliberate and fluid body movements designed to slow and focus the mind and breathing to foster a greater sense of health and wellbeing

Tai Chi Health Society Riverdale Georgia 770-994-0759

Tassili's Raw Reality—Astonishing Raw Food Restaurant located at 1059 Ralph David Abernathy Atlanta Ga. 30310
http://www.tassilisrawreality.com/

Toxic Substances in the Home—Chemicals such as bleach, detergents, bath and window cleaners, radon gas and unventilated fumes that can be harmful when exposed to the body

Thymus Thumping—The tapping of the thymus gland, an organ located at the base of the neck associated with the immune system, in order to promote a healthy immune response

Yoga—A system or set of breathing exercises, stretches and postures derived from or based on Hindu yoga practiced to promote unity of mind, body and spirit

ABOUT THE AUTHOR

Charise—empowered became Chi Ma'at! Living in Georgia, practicing Tai Chi and now working at *Tassili's Raw Reality*, the astounding and incomparable Raw Food Restaurant! Chi Ma'at can be contacted at footprinz1@yahoo.com

Cover photo—taken from youtube video. This is the Best video regarding the year 2012. Little Grandmother Shaman Keisha.

~ Write your own healing journey here! ~

❧ Write your own healing journey here! ☙

❦ Write your own healing journey here! ❦

❧ Write your own healing journey here! ☙

Write your own healing journey here!

❧ Write your own healing journey here! ☙

Write your own healing journey here!

❦ Write your own healing journey here! ❦

❧ Write your own healing journey here! ❧

❧ Write your own healing journey here! ☙

◈ Write your own healing journey here! ◈

❧ Write your own healing journey here! ❧

❧ Write your own healing journey here! ❦

✍ Write your own healing journey here! ✍

❧ Write your own healing journey here! ❧

❧ Write your own healing journey here! ☙

❧ Write your own healing journey here! ☙

❦ Write your own healing journey here! ❦

❧ Write your own healing journey here! ☙

❧ Write your own healing journey here! ☙

❧ Write your own healing journey here! ❧

❧ Write your own healing journey here! ☙

Write your own healing journey here!

Write your own healing journey here!

Write your own healing journey here!